Chemo Jou

Chemotherapy Treatment Cycle Tracker, Side Effects Journal & Medical Appointments Diary, 8" x 10", Over 165 Pages, Notebook

by Anthea Peries

Version 1.0 – June 2018

Published by Anthea Peries

ISBN-13: 978-1722188146

DISCLAIMER

This book contains the ideas and opinions of the author. It is intended to provide information material on the subject addressed in the book. It is sold with the understanding that the author is not engaged in rendering medical, health, psychological or any kind of personal, professional services. If the reader requires personal medical or other health advice/assistance, competent professional should be consulted. The author specifically disclaims all responsibility, loss, or risk, personal or otherwise, that is incurred directly or indirectly, of the use and application of any of the content of this book.

ABOUT THIS BOOK

Chemotherapy treatment is planned by a cancer doctor who will explain the aims of the treatment and possible side effects. Your oncology doctor will ask you to sign a form agreeing to treatment and may talk to you about chemotherapy clinical trials. You may also see an oncology nurse and a pharmacist.

Chemotherapy is usually given to patients as several sessions of treatment, with rest periods in between. Chemotherapy and the rest period make up one cycle of your treatment. Your cancer doctor will explain the number of cycles you need. Sometimes treatment involves having chemotherapy in more than one way, and this should be explained to you by the doctor.

If your chemotherapy treatment plan needs to be changed, your cancer doctor or nurse will explain the reason why. It may be because of the effects of the chemotherapy on your body or on cancer itself. This varies from person to person, for example, your doctor may delay your chemotherapy for a short while, reduce the dose or perhaps put you on a different chemotherapy drug. Your cancer doctor and nurse will monitor you closely during treatment, and they will find it useful if you can provide them with your own feedback using the information you record in this journal. It saves having to remember details from memory.

This journal will enable you to accurately document and regularly monitor how you are feeling; your mood and symptoms during your chemotherapy cycles and rest periods. For example, you can record mood, side effects, sugar levels if diabetic and temperature. By completing each chart per cycle you will start to see trends and patterns to help manage and raise awareness on how your body reacts to the treatment, and you can share any information with your doctor and nurse if you wish. This decorative 8" x 10" journal contains up to 8 cycle charts in landscape, each consisting of 21 days per cycle. There are examples of how to complete the simple table charts at the beginning of each chart.

If you have cancer or know someone who does, this journal is a useful gift and self-monitoring tool used in conjunction as a personal diary, to record any type of oncology journey. The charts will assist in jotting down quick notes with ample space to record greater details, facts, thoughts and doodles. There are positive, uplifting quotes to reflect on during rest periods with an 'appointments' and 'dates to remember' section to remind you about medical and other appointments.

There are twelve calming images to colour in using colouring pencils at the back of this book as a bonus. Paying attention to the present moment by colouring in beautiful illustrations and inspirational words can help improve your well-being; feel relaxed, calm and less anxious when emotionally upset and stressed. Let positive words sink into your sub-conscious mind to help support your state of mind to a higher level. Attentively and creatively colouring in peaceful images will enable you to focus on wonderful, vibrant colours.

Dedicated to my beloved father

APPOINTMENTS

WEEK 1	MONDAY	TUESDAY	WEDNESDAY	THURSDAY	FRIDAY

WEEK 2	MONDAY	TUESDAY	WEDNESDAY	THURSDAY	FRIDAY

WEEK 3	MONDAY	TUESDAY	WEDNESDAY	THURSDAY	FRIDAY

WEEK 4	MONDAY	TUESDAY	WEDNESDAY	THURSDAY	FRIDAY

APPOINTMENTS

WEEK 5	MONDAY	TUESDAY	WEDNESDAY	THURSDAY	FRIDAY

WEEK 6	MONDAY	TUESDAY	WEDNESDAY	THURSDAY	FRIDAY

WEEK 7	MONDAY	TUESDAY	WEDNESDAY	THURSDAY	FRIDAY

WEEK 8	MONDAY	TUESDAY	WEDNESDAY	THURSDAY	FRIDAY

DATES TO REMEMBER

DATE	EVENT	DATE	EVENT

CYCLE 1	DAY	DATE	BLOOD COUNT LOW/HIGH	MOOD, SIDE EFFECTS & COMMENTS	SOLUTION	Sugar level mmol	Temp C
Example: CYCLE 1	Example: DAY 1	Example: 1st January 2016	Example: blood count drops or rises.	Example: nausea/vomiting, dizzy, fatigue, rash, pain, breathless, loss of appetite, constipation, diarrhoea, fever, loss of hair, sore / dry mouth, depressed or duration of treatment and type.	Example: sip of water, rest, eat.	Example: 5.4	Example: 36.7
CYCLE 1	DAY 1						
	DAY 2						
	DAY 3						
	DAY 4						
	DAY 5						
	DAY 6						
	DAY 7						
	DAY 8						
	DAY 9						
	DAY 10						
	DAY 11						
	DAY 12						
	DAY 13						
	DAY 14						
	DAY 15						
	DAY 16						
	DAY 17						
	DAY 18						
	DAY 19						
	DAY 20						
	DAY 21						

FURTHER NOTES

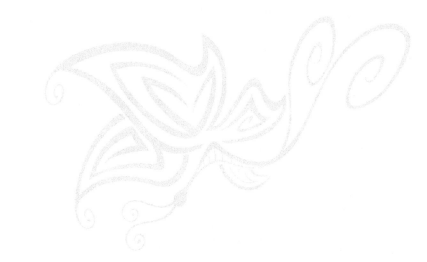

Feelings, thoughts & doodles

Know yourself.

CYCLE 2	DAY	DATE	BLOOD COUNT LOW/HIGH	MOOD, SIDE EFFECTS & COMMENTS	SOLUTION	Sugar level mmol	Temp C
Example: CYCLE 2	Example: DAY 1	Example: 1st January 2016	Example: blood count drops or rises.	Example: nausea/vomiting, dizzy, fatigue, rash, pain, breathless, loss of appetite, constipation, diarrhoea, fever, loss of hair, sore / dry mouth, depressed or duration of treatment and type.	Example: sip of water, rest, eat.	Example: 5.4	Example: 36.7
CYCLE 2	DAY 1						
	DAY 2						
	DAY 3						
	DAY 4						
	DAY 5						
	DAY 6						
	DAY 7						
	DAY 8						
	DAY 9						
	DAY 10						
	DAY 11						
	DAY 12						
	DAY 13						
	DAY 14						
	DAY 15						
	DAY 16						
	DAY 17						
	DAY 18						
	DAY 19						
	DAY 20						
	DAY 21						

FURTHER NOTES

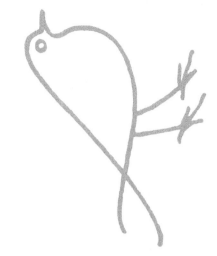

Thoughts & doodles

The point of power is always in the present moment.

CYCLE 3	DAY	DATE	BLOOD COUNT LOW/HIGH	MOOD, SIDE EFFECTS & COMMENTS	SOLUTION	Sugar level mmol	Temp C
Example: CYCLE 3	*Example: DAY 1*	*Example: 1st January 2016*	*Example: blood count drops or rises.*	*Example: nausea/vomiting, dizzy, fatigue, rash, pain, breathless, loss of appetite, constipation, diarrhoea, fever, loss of hair, sore / dry mouth, depressed or duration of treatment and type.*	*Example: sip of water, rest, eat.*	*Example: 5.4*	*Example: 36.7*
CYCLE 3	DAY 1						
	DAY 3						
	DAY 4						
	DAY 5						
	DAY 6						
	DAY 7						
	DAY 8						
	DAY 9						
	DAY 10						
	DAY 11						
	DAY 12						
	DAY 13						
	DAY 14						
	DAY 15						
	DAY 16						
	DAY 17						
	DAY 18						
	DAY 19						
	DAY 20						
	DAY 21						

FURTHER NOTES

Thoughts & doodles

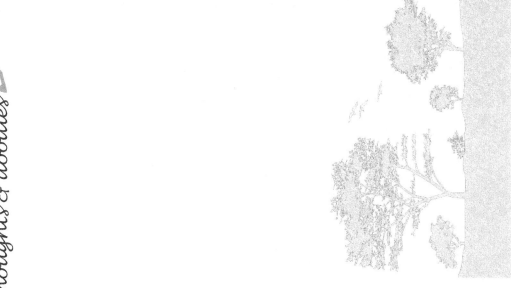

Love is all that matters in
this world.

CYCLE 4	DAY	DATE	BLOOD COUNT LOW/HIGH	MOOD, SIDE EFFECTS & COMMENTS	SOLUTION	Sugar level mmol	Temp C
Example: CYCLE 4	Example: DAY 1	Example: 1st January 2016	Example: blood count drops or rises.	Example: nausea/vomiting, dizzy, fatigue, rash, pain, breathless, loss of appetite, constipation, diarrhoea, fever, loss of hair, sore / dry mouth, depressed or duration of treatment and type.	Example: sip of water, rest, eat.	Example: 5.4	Example: 36.7
CYCLE 4	DAY 1						
	DAY 2						
	DAY 3						
	DAY 4						
	DAY 5						
	DAY 6						
	DAY 7						
	DAY 8						
	DAY 9						
	DAY 10						
	DAY 11						
	DAY 12						
	DAY 13						
	DAY 14						
	DAY 15						
	DAY 16						
	DAY 17						
	DAY 18						
	DAY 19						
	DAY 20						
	DAY 21						

FURTHER NOTES

Thoughts & doodles

Look within to find your

treasures.

CYCLE 5	DATE	BLOOD COUNT LOW/HIGH	MOOD, SIDE EFFECTS & COMMENTS	SOLUTION	Sugar level mmol	Temp C
Example: CYCLE 5	Example: 1st January 2016	Example: blood count drops or rises.	Example: nausea/vomiting, dizzy, fatigue, rash, pain, breathless, loss of appetite, constipation, diarrhoea, fever, loss of hair, sore / dry mouth, depressed or duration of treatment and type.	Example: sip of water, rest, eat.	Example: 5.4	Example: 36.7
CYCLE 5 DAY 1						
DAY 2						
DAY 3						
DAY 4						
DAY 5						
DAY 6						
DAY 7						
DAY 8						
DAY 9						
DAY 10						
DAY 11						
DAY 12						
DAY 13						
DAY 14						
DAY 15						
DAY 16						
DAY 17						
DAY 18						
DAY 19						
DAY 20						
DAY 21						

FURTHER NOTES

Thoughts & doodles

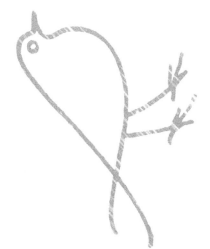

Accept and acknowledge your feelings whether positive or negative.

CYCLE 6		DATE	BLOOD COUNT LOW/HIGH	MOOD, SIDE EFFECTS & COMMENTS	SOLUTION	Sugar level mmol	Temp C
Example: CYCLE 6	Example: DAY 1	Example: 1st January 2016	Example: blood count drops or rises.	Example: nausea/vomiting, dizzy, fatigue, rash, pain, breathless, loss of appetite, constipation, diarrhoea, fever, loss of hair, sore / dry mouth, depressed or duration of treatment and type.	Example: sip of water, rest, eat.	Example: 5.4	Example: 36.7
CYCLE 6	DAY 1						
	DAY 2						
	DAY 3						
	DAY 4						
	DAY 5						
	DAY 6						
	DAY 7						
	DAY 8						
	DAY 9						
	DAY 10						
	DAY 11						
	DAY 12						
	DAY 13						
	DAY 14						
	DAY 15						
	DAY 16						
	DAY 17						
	DAY 18						
	DAY 19						
	DAY 20						
	DAY 21						

FURTHER NOTES

Thoughts & doodles

Rely on Divine guidance and wisdom to protect you at all times.

CYCLE 7	DATE	BLOOD COUNT LOW/HIGH	MOOD, SIDE EFFECTS & COMMENTS	SOLUTION	Sugar level mmol	Temp C
Example: CYCLE 7	Example: 1st January 2016	Example: blood count drops or rises.	Example: nausea/vomiting, dizzy, fatigue, rash, pain, breathless, loss of appetite, constipation, diarrhoea, fever, loss of hair, sore / dry mouth, depressed or duration of treatment and type.	Example: sip of water, rest, eat.	Example: 5.4	Example: 36.7
CYCLE 7						
DAY 1						
DAY 2						
DAY 3						
DAY 4						
DAY 5						
DAY 6						
DAY 7						
DAY 8						
DAY 9						
DAY 10						
DAY 11						
DAY 12						
DAY 13						
DAY 14						
DAY 15						
DAY 16						
DAY 17						
DAY 18						
DAY 19						
DAY 20						
DAY 21						

FURTHER NOTES

Thoughts & doodles

create peacefulness in
your mind and trust your
inner wisdom.

CYCLE 8	DATE	BLOOD COUNT LOW/HIGH	MOOD, SIDE EFFECTS & COMMENTS	SOLUTION	Sugar level mmol	Temp C
Example: CYCLE 8	Example: 1st January 2016	Example: blood count drops or rises.	Example: nausea/vomiting, dizzy, fatigue, rash, pain, breathless, loss of appetite, constipation, diarrhoea, fever, loss of hair, sore / dry mouth, depressed or duration of treatment and type.	Example: sip of water, rest, eat.	Example: 5.4	Example: 36.7
Example: DAY 1						
CYCLE 8	DAY 1					
	DAY 2					
	DAY 3					
	DAY 4					
	DAY 5					
	DAY 6					
	DAY 7					
	DAY 8					
	DAY 9					
	DAY 10					
	DAY 11					
	DAY 12					
	DAY 13					
	DAY 14					
	DAY 15					
	DAY 16					
	DAY 17					
	DAY 18					
	DAY 19					
	DAY 20					
	DAY 21					

FURTHER NOTES

Thoughts & doodles

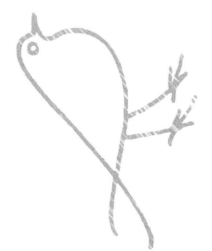

Believe in yourself at all times.

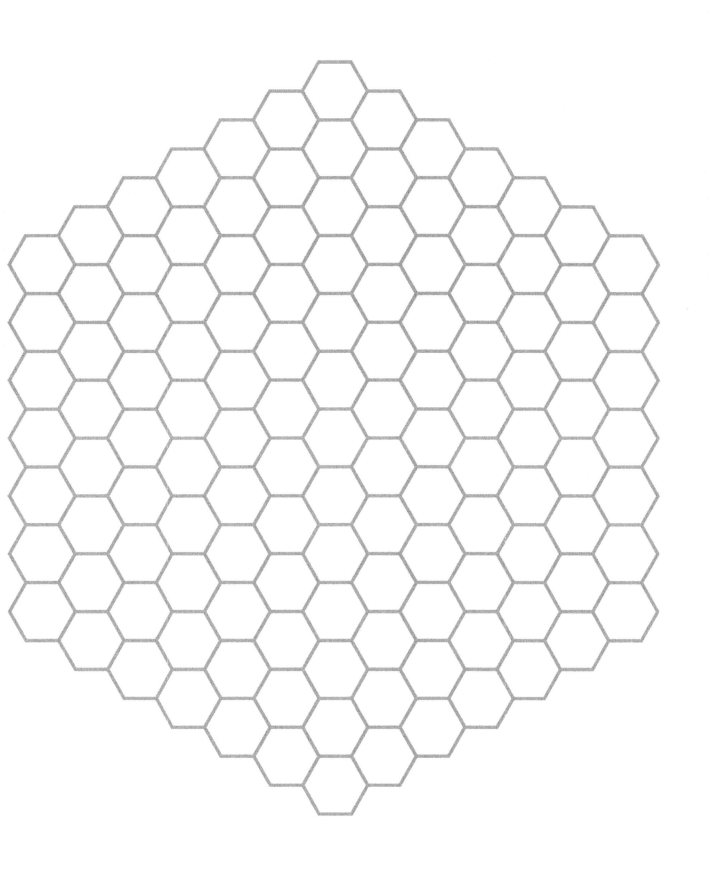

NOTES

NOTES

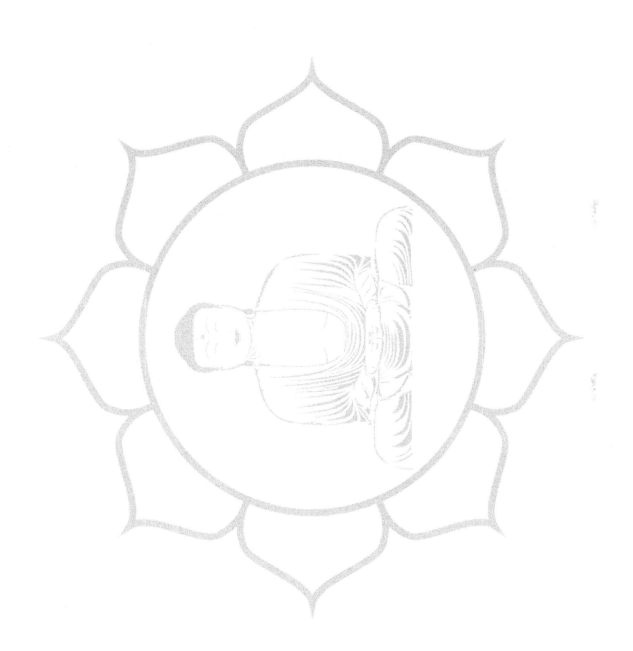

NOTES

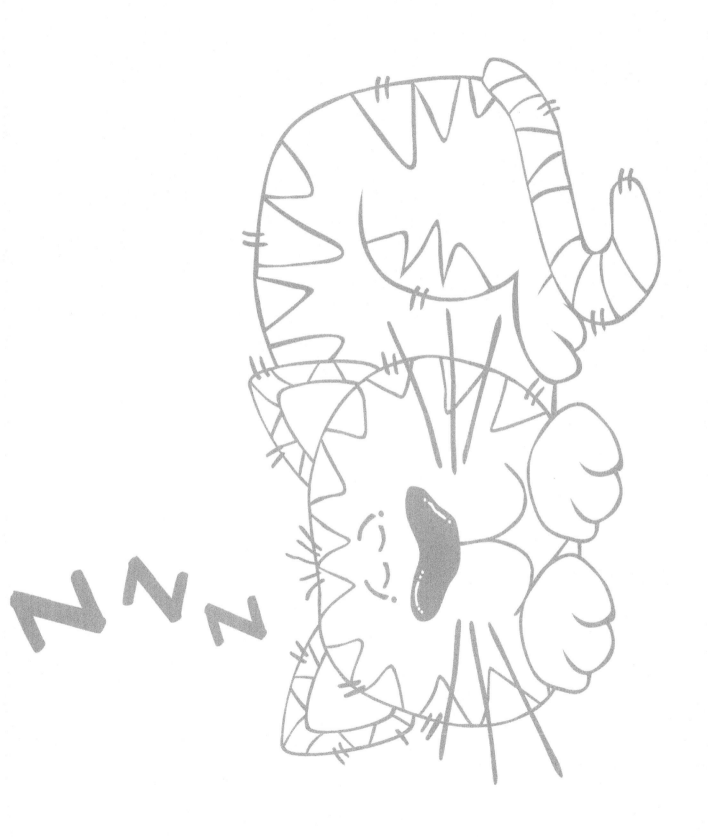

NOTES

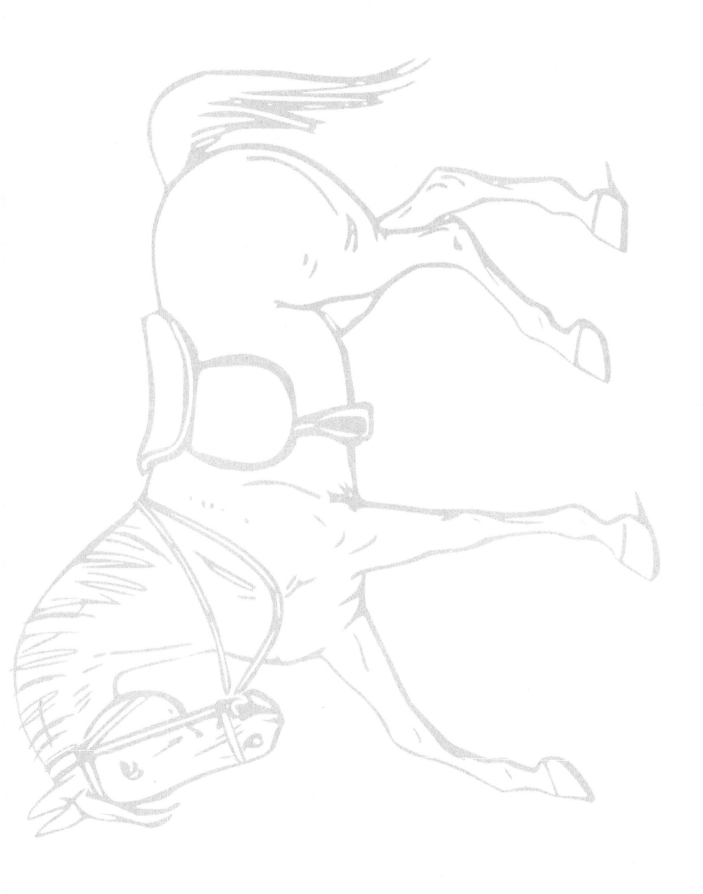

NOTES

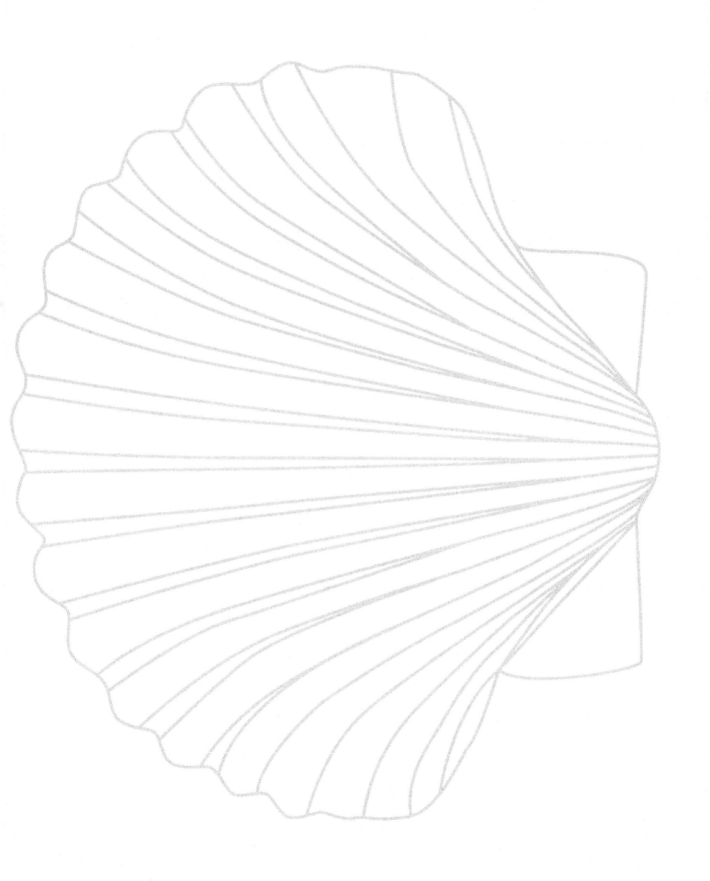

NOTES

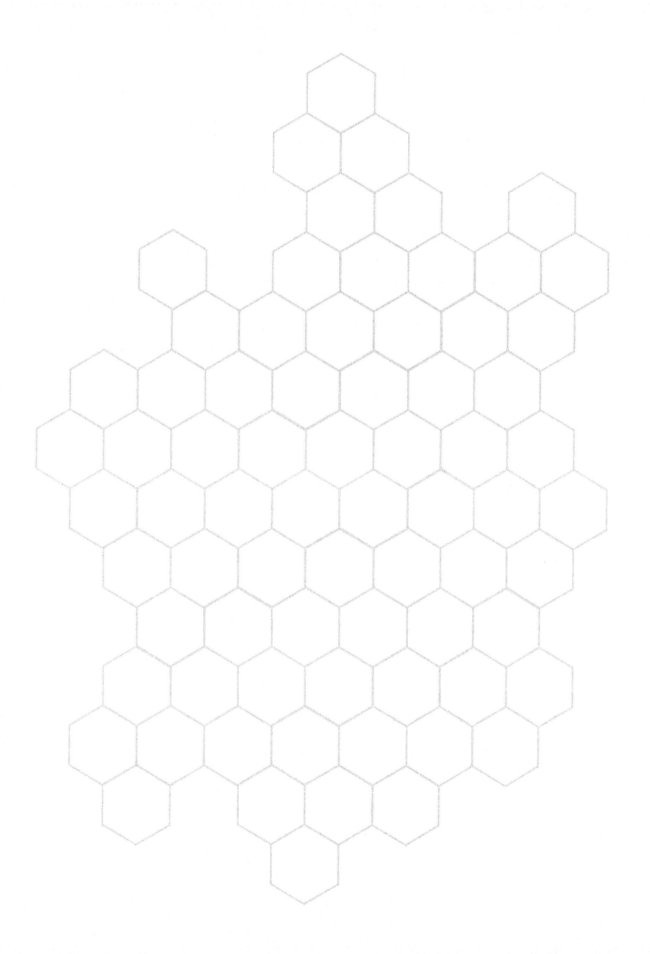

NOTES

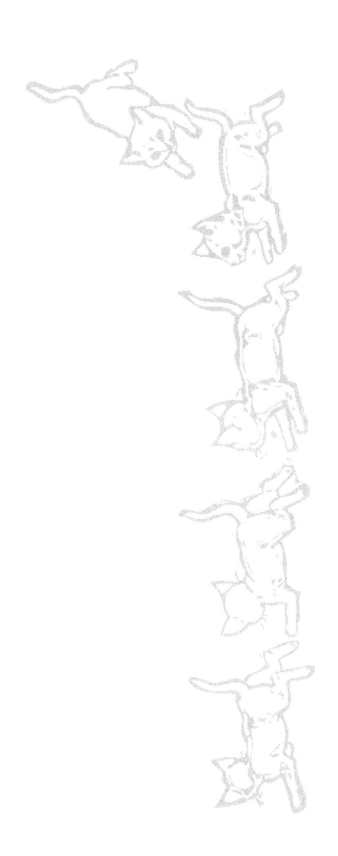

NOTES

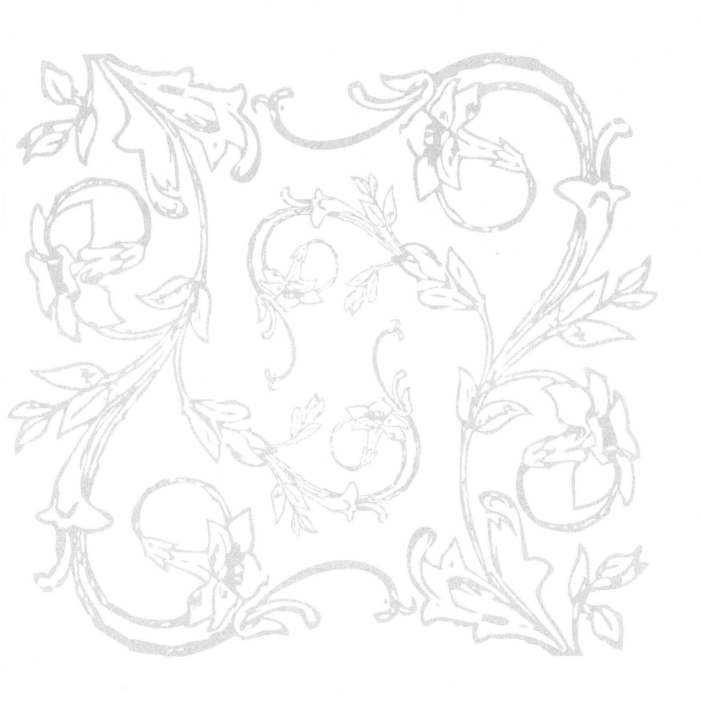

NOTES

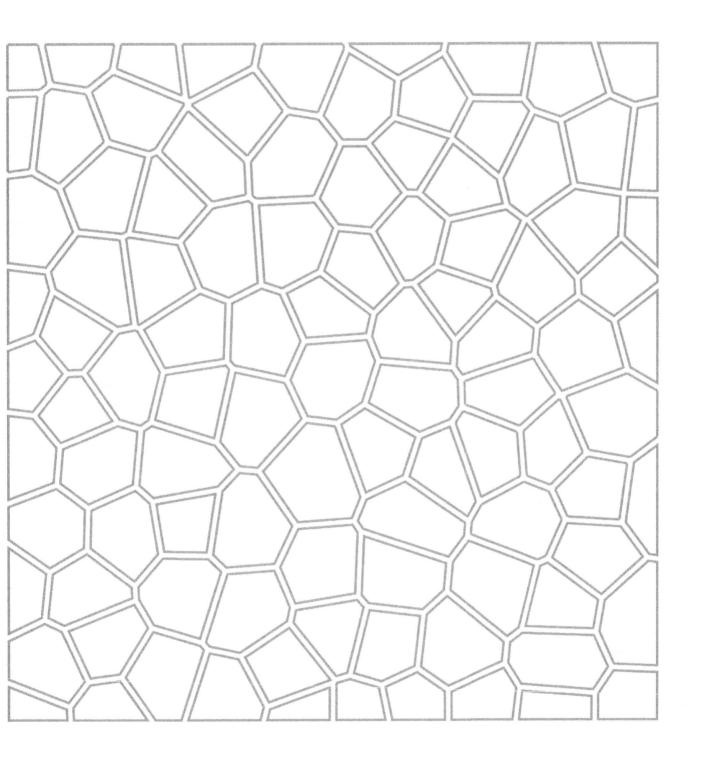

NOTES

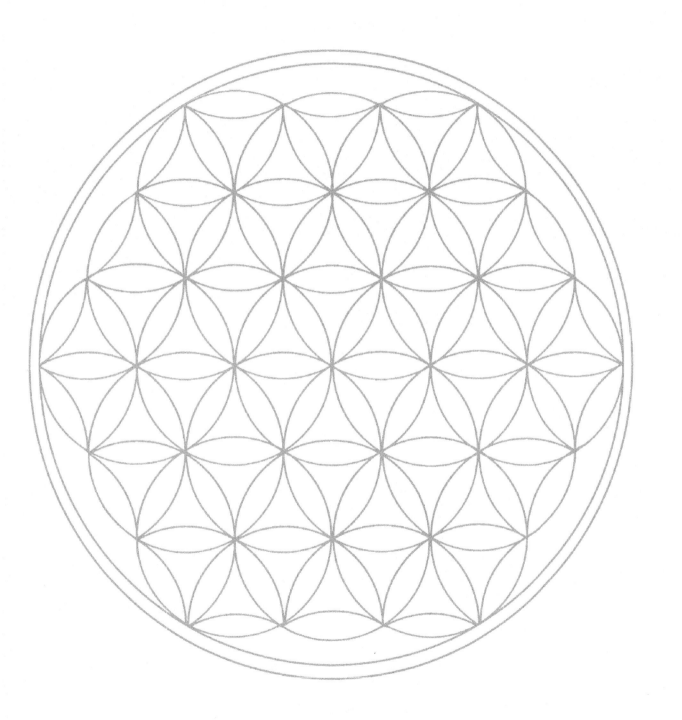

NOTES

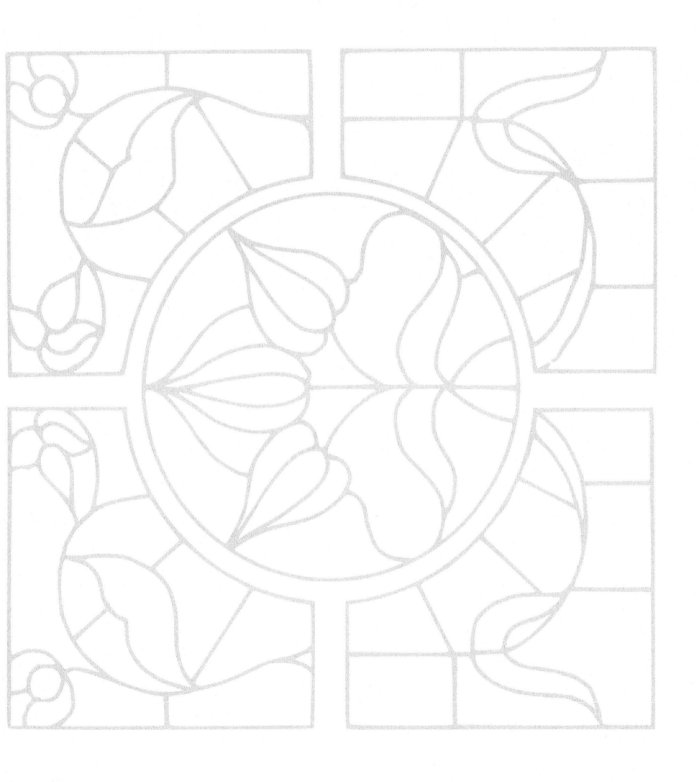

ABOUT THE AUTHOR

Anthea Peries BSc (Hons) completed her undergraduate studies in several branches of the sciences including Biology, Brain and Behaviour and Child Development; a former member of the British Psychological Society. She has experience in counselling and is a former senior management executive. Born and bred in London, Anthea enjoys fine cuisine, writing, and has travelled most of the world. She lives in the United Kingdom and has an extremely spoilt cat named Giorgio.

Thank you for buying this book. If you found the information helpful please leave an honest review – your feedback is valued and it may help someone.

Made in United States
North Haven, CT
17 January 2022